FREESTYLE 2018

Quick and Easy Recipes, a Complete Guide for WEIGHT LOSS

2018
DANIEL ROSS
GAT

Text Copyright © Daniel Ross

Legal & Disclaimer

The information contained in this book and its contents is not designed to replace or take the place of any form of medical or professional advice; and is not meant to replace the need for independent medical, financial, legal or other professional advice or services, as may be required. The content and information in this book has been provided for educational and entertainment purposes only.

The content and information contained in this book has been compiled from sources deemed reliable, and it is accurate to the best of the Author's knowledge, information and belief. However, the Author cannot guarantee its accuracy and validity and cannot be held liable for any errors and/or omissions. Further, changes are periodically made to this book as and when needed. Where appropriate and/or necessary, you must consult a professional (including but not limited to your doctor, attorney, financial advisor or such other professional advisor) before using any of the suggested remedies, techniques, or information in this book.

Upon using the contents and information contained in this book, you agree to hold harmless the Author from and against any damages, costs, and expenses, including any legal fees potentially resulting from the application of any of the information provided by this book. This disclaimer applies to any loss, damages or injury caused by the use and application, whether directly or indirectly, of any advice or information presented, whether for breach of contract, tort, negligence, personal injury, criminal intent, or under any other cause of action.

You agree to accept all risks of using the information presented inside this book.

You agree that by continuing to read this book, where appropriate and/or necessary, you shall consult a professional (including but not limited to your doctor, attorney, or financial advisor or such other advisor as needed) before using any of the suggested remedies, techniques, or information in this book.

Introduction

"You are what you eat"

For years our recipes have based its knowledge on exclusively scientific approaches on correct weight regulation. This book is a large collection of unique recipes for the preparation of delicious and useful recipes for perfectly proper nutrition, the use of which will also help you correctly use mostly any healthy diet program.

The main feature of this book is that you no longer need to constantly think out how to make healthy food tasty. Often in life, healthy food and tasty food are different concepts. In this case, the question arises: how is it possible to lose weight, but at the same time to eat deliciously, using your preferences in food and products?

The book contains 4 most common cooking recipe groups, namely:

Starters and Light Meals
Salads—Sides and Main
Soups—Starters and Main Dishes
Beef, Pork, and Lamb

We offer these groups because they are commonly used mostly any day in any kitchen, so you don't have to change your cooking preferences. With the help of our recipes, you can easily prepare a variety of dishes and immediately see their complete nutritional content, which will help you avoid an overabundance of calories throughout the day.

Be sure to remember that eating is 80% of success in the process of losing weight, and the remaining 20% is an active way of life. In order for both of these factors to work for you, you need to follow the chosen weight loss plan and set achievable goals. Say you want to lose 10% of a current weight and this is an achievable goal. So your next step should be healthy cooking and active way of life. As soon as you will see the results, set your next goal and become a go-getter with our recipes!

Table of Contents

STARTERS and LIGHT MEALS

Classic Guacamole Jamie

Serve guacamole on a plate with fresh vegetables, finely chopped pieces of zucchini and cucumber, add a few rings of sweet pepper and halves of radish. Put it on the leaves of chicory salad and densely sliced pieces of white mushrooms.

Ingredients (6 serves):

Large Hass avocado, halved and pitted	1
Plum tomatoes, chopped	2
Small onion, chopped	½
Cup chopped fresh cilantro	¼
Small jalapeño pepper, seeded and minced	1
Lime juice	1 tablespoon
Salt	½ teaspoon
Black pepper	¼ teaspoon

Directions:

1. Using a spoon, separate the pulp from the rind.

2. Chop it to a pulp-like mass,

3. Add all the remaining elements and mix to a single mass. You can serve the dish to the table immediately, and if you cook in advance, cover it with the food stretch to avoid airing. Store at room temperature and serve within 2 hours.

PER SERVING (¼ cup): 59 grams, 58 Cal, 5 g Total Fat, 1 g Sat Fat, 0 g Trans Fat, 0 mg Chol, 200 mg Sod, 4 g Total Carb, 1 g Total Sugar, 2 g Fib, 1 g Prot, 6 mg Calc.

Classic and tasty Baba Ghanoush

Add a natural smoky flavor to the eggplant, then soak 1 cup of hickory or apple wood chips in water for 30 minutes. Drain the water off and pour the soaked chips on the hot coals, in case you are using a charcoal grill. If you cook on a gas grill, then pour the soaked wood chips on a small disposable iron foil with holes, put it on the top of the gas grill and cook the eggplant as indicated in the recipe.

Ingredients (8 serves):

Eggplant	1 (1-pound)
Lemon juice	3 tablespoons
Tahini	2 tablespoons
Extra-virgin olive oil	1 tablespoon
Garlic cloves, minced	2
Salt	¾ teaspoon
Black pepper	¼ teaspoon

Directions:

1. Preheat the oven to 400 ° F. Lay foil over the baking form and spray using a non-stick spray.

2. Pierce the eggplant with a knife in several places and lay it on the baking sheet. Bake the eggplant for 45 minutes turning it over from time to time, until it becomes soft.

3. Remove the eggplant and put it on the plate to cool. When the eggplant has cooled, peel the skin off with a knife and cut it into slices. Put the eggplant in a blender and grind it to a puree-like mass. Add all the remaining ingredients and mix again into a single mass. Serve immediately after cooking, or pack in a food container and store in a freezer for up to 4 days.

PER SERVING (¼ cup): 59 grams, 52 Cal, 4 g Total Fat, 1 g Sat Fat, 0 g Trans Fat, 0 mg Chol, 221 mg Sod, 5 g Total Carb, 2 g Total Sugar, 1 g Fib, 1 g Prot, 11 mg Calc.

Roasted Red Pepper Dip

If you are in a hurry and have almost no time for cooking, use a 7-ounce jar of fried pepper canned in water. Pour the liquid into a container and place the peppers on a plate. Continue to follow the recipe and if the sauce turns too thick add a small amount of liquid in which the peppers were packed.

Ingredients (4 serves):
Large red bell peppers

Extra-virgin olive oil	1 tablespoon
Tomato paste	2 tablespoon
Balsamic vinegar	2 teaspoons
Garlic clove (minced)	1
Salt	½ teaspoon
Black pepper	⅛ teaspoon
Cayenne pepper	⅛ teaspoon

Directions:
1. Cover the broiler pan with foil and preheat it in the oven.

2. Bell pepper must be cut into 2 pieces and then remove the seeds. Put the pepper on broiler pan with the cut side down and cook for about 10 minutes. When the pepper skin is blackened, remove it and put it in a food bag and zip it so it is steamed for about 10 minutes.

3. When the pepper cools and can be taken by hand, peel it and cut into large pieces. Then put it into the food processor and grind it to a puree. Then add the remaining ingredients and stir again until single mass. Serve to the table at once or put in a zip-close plastic container and store up to 4 days.

PER SERVING (¼ cup): 92 grams, 58 Cal, 4 g Total Fat, 1 g Sat Fat, 0 g Trans Fat, 0 mg Chol, 295 mg Sod, 7 g Total Carb, 3 g Total Sugar, 2 g Fib, 1 g Prot, 10 mg Calc.

Sicilian Fried Caponata with an eggplant

Sicilian Caponata dish can be stored in the refrigerator for a long time and keeps all its wonderful taste qualities. Thaw the Caponata correctly and keep its taste, leave it overnight in the fridge or put it on a plate and leave at room temperature.

Ingredients (12 serves):

Olive oil	1 tablespoon
Onion (chopped)	1
Garlic cloves (minced)	3
Celery stalks (diced)	2
Small eggplant (peeled and diced)	1
Water	$^{1}/_{3}$ cup
Large tomato (chopped)	1
Golden raisins	2 tablespoons
Capers (drained)	1 tablespoon
Salt	¾ teaspoon
Black pepper	¼ teaspoon
Pitted green olives (sliced)	8
Large fresh basil leaves (thinly sliced)	4

Directions:

1. Pour some oil into a frying pan and heat it over medium heat. Add chopped garlic and onion and fry for about 5 minutes stirring, until the onion is soft. Add chopped celery and fry it for no more than 4 minutes until it is soft.

2. Cut the eggplant, add it to a skillet, pour water and cook for about 5 minutes. Stirring add tomatoes, raisins, capers and sprinkle with salt and pepper. Stir it from time to time and cook for about 10 minutes. Then remove the lid and cook until the eggplant is soft for about 4 minutes.

3. Remove the frying pan from the plate, add the basil and olives and mix. Then let it cool to room temperature. You can serve the dish to the table immediately or pack it in a food container and store it in the freezer for up to 3 days.

PER SERVING (about ¼ cup): 70 grams, 39 Cal, 2 g Total Fat, 0 g Sat Fat, 0 g Trans Fat, 0 mg Chol, 251 mg Sod, 6 g Total Carb, 3 g Total Sugar, 1 g Fib, 1 g Prot, 11 mg Calc.

Fried Multi Cheese Crisps

In Italy, these amazing and wonderful treats are usually called frico. Traditionally they are cooked with Parmesan cheese only, but in our recipe, we suggest trying a combination of different cheeses and experiencing a unique taste.

Ingredients (8 serves):

Shredded part-skim mozzarella cheese	1 cup
Grated Parmesan cheese	3 tablespoons
All-purpose flour	1 tablespoon
Dried thyme (crumbled Pinch cayenne)	½ teaspoon

Directions:

1. Preheat your oven to a temperature of 400 °F and spray some olive oil on baking sheets.

2. Mix all the ingredients in the bowl. Drop the mixture about 2 inches apart onto the prepared and preheated baking sheet. Continue to bake for about 5 minutes until the cheese in the chips melts and is lightly fried at the edges.

3. Let the crisps to cool for about 1 minute on the baking sheet. Using pancake spatula, transfer the finished chips to a double layer of food paper and allow to cool. Cooked chips are stored up to several days at room temperature.

PER SERVING (2 crisps): 17 grams, 48 Cal, 3 g Total Fat, 2 g Sat Fat, 0 g Trans Fat, 10 mg Chol, 101 mg Sod, 1 g Total Carb, 1 g Total Sugar, 0 g Fib, 4 g Prot, 119 mg Calc.

Italian-Style Stuffed Mushrooms

Put these stuffed mushrooms on the central place of an antipasto plate with grilled vegetables: cherry tomato skewers, radicchio wedges, zucchini slices and grilled Belgian endive.

Ingredients (6 serves):

Sweet Italian turkey sausages, casings removed	½ pound
Cremini mushrooms (about 1½ pounds), stems finely chopped	30
Small onion, finely chopped	1
Garlic clove, minced	1
Chopped fresh parsley	¼ cup
Plain dried bread crumbs	¼ cup
Grated Romano cheese	¼ cup
Large egg white	1
Dried oregano	½ teaspoon
Salt	¼ teaspoon
Black pepper	1/8 teaspoon

Directions:

1. Prepare the oven to 350 °F. Use the non-stick spray on the jelly-roll pan.

2. Now you need to prepare the mushroom filling itself. To do this, put the sausages in a small frying pan and set to an average temperature. Fry them for about 5 minutes stirring with a spatula until they are fried and look no longer pink.

3. Add mushrooms, garlic, and onions and continue stirring for about 6 minutes until the mushrooms turn brown. After transferring everything into a bowl and allow to cool for 5 minutes.

4. Add all the remaining ingredients by mixing them well. Use a teaspoon to fill each mushroom cap with the mixture obtained. Then put all the mushrooms in a prepared

frying pan and bake them about 20 minutes until the mushrooms become soft and filling is heated through. Serve should be warm or hot.

PER SERVING (5 stuffed mushrooms): 92 grams, 91 Cal, 4 g Total Fat, 1 g Sat Fat, 0 g Trans Fat, 19 mg Chol, 355 mg Sod, 7 g Total Carb, 1 g Total Sugar, 1 g Fib, 8 g Prot, 34 mg Calc.

Roasted Vegetable Crostini

This is a delicious mix with a very refined taste. You can also replace some ingredients such as fennel, radicchio or yellow pepper with vegetables that you like more and in equal quantities.

Ingredients (12 serves):

Eggplant (cut into ½-inch dice)	1
Red bell peppers (finely chopped)	2
Zucchini (finely chopped)	2
Onion (sliced)	1
Extra-virgin olive oil	2 tablespoons
Dried oregano	1 teaspoon
Salt	¾ teaspoon
Black pepper	¼ teaspoon
Italian bread, cut into 24 thin slices and toasted	8 ounces
Chopped fresh basil	½ cup
Pitted Kalamata olives, halved	12
Grated Parmesan cheese	¼ cup

Directions:

1. Preheat your oven up to 425 ° F

2. Lay the bell paper, eggplant, zucchini, oregano in a large skillet and season with salt and pepper. Fry the mixture for about 45 minutes stirring occasionally until all ingredients are browned on edges. Then let the mixture to cool to room temperature.

3. Mix the mixture and spoon it evenly onto toasts or tartlets. Sprinkle top with Parmesan, olives, and basil.

PER SERVING (2 crostini): 136 grams, 149 Cal, 5 g Total Fat, 1 g Sat Fat, 0 g Trans Fat, 1 mg Chol, 417 mg Sod, 22 g Total Carb, 4 g Total Sugar, 3 g Fib, 4 g Prot, 62 mg Calc.

White Bean Bruschetta

Sprinkle finely chopped basil onto each bruschetta with chopped fresh tomato.

Ingredients (4 serves):

Can cannellini (white kidney) beans, rinsed and drained	1
Chopped fresh flat-leaf parsley	2 tablespoons
Zest and juice of lemon	2 tablespoons
Extra-virgin olive oil	2 teaspoons
Salt	¼ teaspoon
Black pepper	¼ teaspoon
Garlic clove, cut in half	1
Thin slices whole wheat Italian bread, toasted	12

Directions:

1. Mix the beans with 1 teaspoon of parsley, add the lemon juice and zest, olive oil, salt, and pepper in a medium-sized bowl.

2. Rub cut the garlic in half and grate each toasted toast on one side. Then, on the grated side of the toast, place the mixture of beans evenly and sprinkle with finely chopped parsley.

PER SERVING (3 bruschettas): 128 grams, 169 Cal, 2 g Total Fat, 1 g Sat Fat, 0 g Trans Fat, 0 mg Chol, 464 mg Sod, 33 g Total Carb, 2 g Total Sugar, 7 g Fib, 7 g Prot, 69 mg Calc.

Smoky Onion Tartlets

In order to caramelize onions, they must be cooked slowly and at medium temperature. During this time, the onion acquires its deep color and shows natural sweetness.

Ingredients (15 serves):

Sweet onions, such as Vidalia (about 1¾ pounds), thinly sliced	2
Smoked paprika	¾ teaspoon
Salt	¾ teaspoon
Black pepper	½ teaspoon
Shredded Gruyère cheese	⅓ cup
Packages frozen mini phyllo pastry shells (30 shells total)	2

Directions:

1. To make a filling, sprinkle a large frying pan with a little oil. Add the onion and fry it for about 25 minutes until it is soft and golden. Add paprika, pepper, and salt. Stir and remove the frying pan from the stove for 15 minutes and let it cool.

2. Preheat oven to 350 ° F

3. Add the Gruyère cheese to the cooled mixture. Lay the test bowls on the baking tray and add 1½ teaspoons of onion mixture to each shell.

4. Put the baking tray in the oven and bake for about 6 minutes until the dough is slightly crispy around the edges and soft in the middle. Serve warm or hot.

PER SERVING (2 tartlets): 26 grams, 51 Cal, 3 g Total Fat, 1 g Sat Fat, 0 g Trans Fat, 3 mg Chol, 150 mg Sod, 5 g Total Carb, 1 g Total Sugar, 0 g Fib, 1 g Prot, 28 mg Calc.

Lemon-Thyme Zucchini on Flatbread

Packages of naan can be easily found in the bread section in supermarkets.

Ingredients (6 serves):

Lemon juice	3 tablespoons
Extra-virgin olive oil 3 garlic cloves, minced	1½ teaspoons
Chopped fresh thyme	2 teaspoons
Salt	½ teaspoon
Zucchini, cut crosswise in half, then lengthwise into ¼-inch slices	2
Whole wheat naan flatbreads	3
Crumbled soft goat cheese, at room temperature	½ cup

Directions:

1. Mix the lemon juice, olive oil, thyme in a large plastic bag with a zip and add salt and zucchini. Press the air out of the bag and turn to coat zucchini. Leave for 30 minutes.

2. Spray the grill with oil. Then heat the grill rack to medium temperature.

3. Put the zucchini on the grill and fry on both sides for about 2 minutes until it becomes tender. Then place the grill on the naan and fry for about 2 minutes until lightly crisp. Spread evenly goat cheese and then zucchini on naan. Close the grill cover for 3 minutes while the naan is slightly charred. Put it on a dish and cut into 4 pieces.

PER SERVING (½ garnished flatbread): 118 grams, 158 Cal, 4 g Total Fat, 1 g Sat Fat, 0 g Trans Fat, 4 mg Chol, 240 mg Sod, 24 g Total Carb, 2 g Total Sugar, 5 g Fib, 8 g Prot, 34 mg Calc.

Tasty Beef Picadillo in Lettuce Leaves

This wonderful mixture of beef can also be perfectly used as stuffing for various vegetables such as baby eggplant, tomatoes, zucchini and bell paper.

Ingredients (8 serves):

Onion, chopped	1
Garlic cloves, minced	2
Lean ground beef (7% fat or less)	1 pound
Sliced pitted green olives	¼ cup
Chili powder	1 tablespoon
Ground cumin	2 teaspoons
Chopped fresh cilantro	¼ cup
Red wine vinegar	2 tablespoons
Salt	¾ teaspoon
Black pepper	¾ teaspoon
Boston lettuce leaves	8

Directions:

1. Spray the frying pan with nonstick spray and preheat on medium heat. Then put onions and fry for about 5 minutes until the onion becomes soft and golden. Add garlic and stir constantly for about 30 seconds until garlic gives a fragrant smell. Add chopped beef, cook the mixture for about 5 minutes and stir constantly with a spatula.

2. After adding olives, cumin and chili powder in a frying pan and cook for about 2 minutes stirring occasionally. Add the vinegar, salt, coriander, pepper, and cook, stirring constantly for about 30 seconds until all the vinegar is evaporated.

3. Lay about $^1/^3$ cup of picadillo on the lettuce leaf and spread it nicely on a large plate.

PER SERVING (1 filled lettuce leaf): 83 grams, 99 Cal, 4 g Total Fat, 1 g Sat Fat, 0 g Trans Fat, 32 mg Chol, 223 mg Sod, 4 g Total Carb, 1 g Total Sugar, 1 g Fib, 12 g Prot, 19 mg Calc.

Garlic Shrimp Tapas

Having cleared the shrimp from the shell, you need to make a cut along the tail of each peeled shrimp with a sharp knife and remove the vein. Rinse the shrimp under running cold water and remove the remaining moisture with paper towels.

Ingredients (8 serves):

Olive oil	1 tablespoon
Garlic cloves, minced	4
Large shrimp (about 1 pound), peeled and deveined	24
Dried oregano	¾ teaspoon
Red pepper flakes	⅛ teaspoon

Directions:

1. Heat oil in a very large nonstick skillet over medium heat. Add garlic and cook, stirring, until fragrant, about 30 seconds. Increase heat to medium-high; add shrimp and sprinkle with oregano and pepper flakes. Cook, stirring, until shrimp are just opaque throughout, about 2 minutes. Serve hot or warm.

2. Pour the oil into a large non-stick frying pan and warm it up at medium temperature. Add garlic to frying pan and cook for about 30 seconds.

3. Then slightly increase the temperature and add shrimps, pepper flakes, and oregano. Cook stirring from time to time for about 2 minutes. It could be served hot or warm.

PER SERVING (3 shrimps): 20 grams, 34 Cal, 2 g Total Fat, 0 g Sat Fat, 0 g Trans Fat, 32 mg Chol, 37 mg Sod, 1 g Total Carb, 0 g Total Sugar, 0 g Fib, 4 g Prot, 12 mg Calc.

SALADS—SIDES and MAIN

Whole Leaf Caesar Salad with Golden Croutons

In order to turn out Caesar salad exceptionally delicious, use only small leaves of romaine lettuce that are inside the rocker.

Ingredients (6 serves):

Cubes (¾-inch) whole grain bread	1 cup
Small garlic clove, peeled	1
Salt	¼ teaspoon
Reduced-sodium chicken broth	3 tablespoons
Grated Parmesan cheese	2 tablespoons
Extra-virgin olive oil	1 tablespoon
Reduced-fat mayonnaise	1 tablespoon
Chopped fresh flat-leaf parsley	1 tablespoon
Cider vinegar	1 tablespoon
Dijon mustard	1 tablespoon
Anchovy paste Pinch black pepper	1 tablespoon
Lightly packed small romaine lettuce leaves	8 cups

Directions:

1 Preheat the oven to 350 ° F.

2 Evenly spread the bread cubes over the non-stick pan and bake for about 10 minutes until golden brown.

3 With the flat side of the knife, grind the peeled garlic and mix with the salt.

4 To prepare the dressing for the salad, mix in a small bowl: broth, olive oil, 1 tablespoon of Parmesan, mayonnaise, mustard, vinegar, anchovy paste, garlic paste, and pepper.

5 Lay the leaves of romaine and croutons in a large salad bowl, then add the dressing to the salad, and mix equally. Put salad on six plates and sprinkle 1 tablespoon of grated cheese on top.

Per serving: (1⅓ cups): 91 grams, 66 Cal, 4 g Total Fat, 1 g Sat Fat, 0 g Trans Fat, 3 mg Chol, 235 mg Sod, 5 g Total Carb, 1 g Total Sugar, 2 g Fib, 3 g Prot, 61 mg Calc.

Beet, Apple, and Watercress Salad

In order to avoid staining the apple beets, put the apple in a container and mix with a small amount of salad dressing, and then lay it over the cooked salad top.

Ingredients (6 serves):

Beets (about 1 pound), trimmed	1 bunch
Granny Smith apple, unpeeled, cored, and diced	1
Watercress, trimmed	1 bunch
Red wine vinegar	3 tablespoons
Olive oil	1 tablespoon
Salt	¼ teaspoon
Black pepper	⅛ teaspoon

Directions:

1 Preheat the oven to 400 ° F.

2 Put the beet on the foil sheet and gently wrap it. Bake beets for about an hour until soft. Open the foil and allow the beet to cool.

3 After the beet has cooled it is necessary to remove the skin from it and cut into cubes. Then mix together apples, watercress, and beets in a salad bowl.

4 To prepare the salad dressing, mix the remaining ingredients thoroughly in a small bowl. Add the dressing to the salad and evenly mix all the ingredients.

Per serving (about ¾ cup): 95 grams, 59 Cal, 2 g Total Fat, 0 g Sat Fat, 0 g Trans Fat, 0 mg Chol, 141 mg Sod, 9 g Total Carb, 6 g Total Sugar, 2 g Fib, 1 g Prot, 24 mg Calc.

Baby Romaine with Clementines and Pecans

If you like Clementine so much, you can use 4 pcs instead of 2

Ingredients (4 serves):

Orange juice	2 tablespoons
Extra-virgin olive oil	2 teaspoons
Salt	¼ teaspoon
Black pepper	¼ teaspoon
Lightly packed baby romaine lettuce	6 cups
Clementines peeled and sectioned	2
Snipped fresh chives	¼ cup
Pecans, chopped and toasted	2 tablespoons

Directions:

1. To prepare the dressing, mix olive oil, salt, a small amount of pepper and orange juice together in a small container. Mix everything evenly with a tablespoon.

2. Toss onions, pecans, and clementines in a salad bowl.

3. Add the dressing to the salad and mix it evenly.

Per serving (about 2 cups): 136 grams, 78 Cal, 5 g Total Fat, 1 g Sat Fat, 0 g Trans Fat, 0 mg Chol, 153 mg Sod, 7 g Total Carb, 5 g Total Sugar, 3 g Fib, 2 g Prot, 42 mg Calc.

Watermelon-Peach Salad with Ricotta Salata

Ricotta salad is obtained by pressing and salting fresh ricotta cheese, and then it is kept for about 2 months. The resulting cheese is somewhat like feta cheese, but with a more refined taste.

Ingredients (4 serves):

Seedless watermelon, rind removed and cut into ¾-inch dice	2-pound piece
Large peaches, pitted and cut into ¾-inch pieces	2
Mini (Persian) cucumbers, thinly sliced	2
Champagne vinegar or white wine vinegar	3 tablespoons
Salt	¼ teaspoon
Coarsely crumbled ricotta salata or feta cheese	½ cup
Scallion (white and light green parts only), cut into very thin strips	1

Directions:

1.Mix together all the ingredients, but for scallion and ricotta in a bowl.

2. let it stand for 10 minutes and then sprinkle the top with scallion and cheese.

3. For a better taste put in a refrigerator for 30 minutes, then mix everything again and put some more cheese on the top.

Per serving (generous 1 cup): 258 grams, 133 Cal, 5 g Total Fat, 3 g Sat Fat, 0 g Trans Fat, 17 mg Chol, 359 mg Sod, 19 g Total Carb, 16 g Total Sugar, 2 g Fib, 4 g Prot, 113 mg Calc.

German Potato Salad with bacon and chopped onion

To make it more crunch double the bell pepper and celery

Ingredients (4 serves):

All-purpose potatoes, peeled 1 onion, finely chopped	1½ pounds
Celery stalk, finely chopped ½ green bell pepper, chopped	1
Bacon, crisp cooked and crumbled	3 slices
Apple juice	½ cup
Cider vinegar	¼ cup
All-purpose flour	1 tablespoon
Salt	½ teaspoon
Black pepper	¼ teaspoon

Directions:

1. First, you need to boil potatoes. To do this, put the peeled potatoes in a bowl and pour water, bring to a boil and reduce the temperature. Cook potatoes for about 20 minutes until soft and then drain.

2. Let the potatoes to cool and cut it into a ¾-inch dice. Mix together onions, potatoes, bell peppers, bacon and potatoes in a salad bowl. Cover with a lid to keep all the ingredients warm.

3 To prepare the dressing, mix together thoroughly, vinegar, apple juice, and flour. Put the mixture in a bowl on the stove, stir constantly and bring to a boil.

4. Reduce the temperature and simmer for about 4 minutes until the mixture becomes thick and add pepper and salt. Then blend thoroughly with the potato mix. Serve the salad warm.

Per serving (about 1 cup): 179 grams, 132 Cal, 2 g Total Fat, 1 g Sat Fat, 0 g Trans Fat, 3 mg Chol, 260 mg Sod, 27 g Total Carb, 5 g Total Sugar, 3 g Fib, 3 g Prot, 26 mg Calc.

Wild Rice Salad with Pecans and Cranberries

In fact, wild rice is a long-grained march grass, which can often be found in the Great Lakes. For commercial purposes, it is also grown in other regions of the United States. The most important thing to remember when cooking wild rice is that you need to cook it until the grains start to open. In case of overcooking, it will become too soft.

Ingredients (8 serves):

Wild rice (about 8 ounces)	1¼ cups
Halved red, green, and/or black grapes	2 cups
Celery stalks with leaves, thinly sliced	2
Chopped fresh flat-leaf parsley	6 tablespoons
Dried cranberries or dried cherries	⅓ cup
Pecans, toasted and chopped	¼ cup
White wine vinegar	2 tablespoons
Extra-virgin olive oil	1 tablespoon
Chopped fresh thyme	1 teaspoon
Salt	¾ teaspoon
Black pepper	½ teaspoon

Directions:

1 Cook the wild rice according to the directions on the package.

2. Drain the remaining water and let cool.

3. Mix all the remaining ingredients in a salad bowl and add the rice.

4. Serve the salad to a table at once or put it in a fridge and serve for 6 hours.

Per serving (¾ cup): 171 grams, 190 Cal, 5 g Total Fat, 1 g Sat Fat, 0 g Trans Fat, 0 mg Chol, 236 mg Sod, 34 g Total Carb, 11 g Total Sugar, 3 g Fib, 5 g Prot, 20 mg Calc.

Wheat Berries with Smoked Turkey and Fruit

Smoked turkey and wheat berries are perfectly combined with peaches, strawberries, and watercress.

Ingredients (4 serves):

Water	2¼ cups
Wheat berries, rinsed	1 cup
Piece smoked turkey, diced	1 (½-pound)
Nectarines, pitted and cut into ½-inch pieces	2
Granny Smith apple, peeled, cored, and diced	1
Red onion, finely chopped	½
Orange juice	¼ cup
Cider vinegar	3 tablespoons
Dijon mustard	1 tablespoon
Honey	1 tablespoon
Baby spinach, coarsely chopped	½ (10-ounce) bag

Directions:

1. Pour the water into a saucepan, bring to a boil and pour the wheat berries.

2. Reduce the temperature and cook for about 1.5 - 2 hours until the wheat berries become soft and the water boils.

3. Then let it cool for about 5 minutes.

4. Mix the turkey, apple, wheat berries, nectarines and vinegar in a large bowl.

5. To prepare salad dressing, mix together the orange juice, mustard, honey, and vinegar in a small container. Season wheat berries and mix evenly.

6. Decorate the plate with spinach leaves and top it with wheat berries mix.

Per serving (2 cups): 296 grams, 322 Cal, 3 g Total Fat, 0 g Sat Fat, 0 g Trans Fat, 24 mg Chol, 673 mg Sod, 62 g Total Carb, 18 g Total Sugar, 10 g Fib, 17 g Prot, 44 mg Calc.

Classic Chicken Salad with fat-free yogurt

Use butter lettuce or Boston leaves to serve the chicken salad.

Ingredients (4 serves):

Plain fat-free yogurt	¼ cup
Reduced-calorie mayonnaise	3 tablespoons
Cider vinegar	1 tablespoon
Dijon mustard	2 teaspoons
Salt	½ teaspoon
Black pepper	¼ teaspoon
Cubed cooked chicken breast	2½ cups
Celery stalks, chopped	2
Grated onion	2 tablespoons

Directions:

1. For salad dressing, combine mayonnaise, mustard, yogurt, vinegar, salt and pepper in a small container.

2. Mix the celery, chicken, and onions in a salad bowl. Add the mixture to yogurt and mix evenly. Cover with a lid and allow to infuse for 1 to 4 hours before serving.

*Per serving (*about 1 cup): 154 grams, 201 Cal, 7 g Total Fat, 2 g Sat Fat, 0 g Trans Fat, 79 mg Chol, 543 mg Sod, 4 g Total Carb, 1 g Total Sugar, 1 g Fib, 29 g Prot, 48 mg Calc

California Seafood Salad

In order to cook the croutons, cut the white bread cut into cubes, then lay them on a baking sheet and spray with olive oil and toss to coat. Preheat the oven to 375 °F and bake them for 6 minutes until they turn golden brown. Let them cool down.

Ingredients (4 serves):

Clam-tomato or tomato juice	¼ cup
Lemon juice	¼ cup
Olive oil	4 teaspoons
Worcestershire sauce	1 tablespoon
Salt	¼ teaspoon
Black pepper	¼ teaspoon
Lightly packed torn red leaf lettuce	4 cups
Cooked crabmeat, picked over	¼ pound
Cooked medium shrimp, peeled and deveined	½ pound
Cherry tomatoes, halved	12
Avocado, pitted, peeled, and diced	½
Navel oranges, peeled and sectioned	½
Croutons	1 cup

Directions:

1 To prepare the dressing, mix lemon juice, oil, clam-tomato juice, Worcester sauce, pepper and salt in a small bowl.

2 Place the leaves of the salad on the dish and crab meat in the middle. Then put the avocado, shrimps, tomatoes, and oranges around the crab meat. Add the dressing to the dish and put the croutons on top.

Per serving (about 2 cups): 328 grams, 261 Cal, 10 g Total Fat, 1 g Sat Fat, 0 g Trans Fat, 141 mg Chol, 562 mg Sod, 23 g Total Carb, 10 g Total Sugar, 6 g Fib, 22 g Prot, 114 mg Calc.

Quinoa-Fruit Salad

Quinoa is a valuable grain crop and the main product of the Incas, which called it the "mother grain". These tiny grains contain the largest amount of protein than any other cereals.

Ingredients (6 serves):

Water	2 cups
Salt	¼ teaspoon
Quinoa, rinsed and drained	1 cup
Chopped fresh mint	⅓cup
Vanilla fat-free yogurt	¼ cup
Orange juice	2 tablespoons
Sliced hulled strawberries	1½ cups
Kiwifruit, peeled and sliced	2
Can mandarin orange sections, drained	1 (11-ounce)

Directions:

1. Pour the water into a saucepan, add salt and bring to a boil. Pour the quinoa into the water and stir. Then reduce the temperature and cook for about 15 minutes, until the quinoa becomes translucent.

2. Mix yogurt, orange juice, and mint to prepare the dressing.

3. Mix kiwi, orange sections, and strawberries in a salad bowl. Fill all ingredients with salad dressing. Then add quinoa, mix everything thoroughly and cover with a lid. Refrigerate the dish for about 2 hours.

Per serving (generous 1 cup): 233 grams, 170 Cal, 2 g Total Fat, 0 g Sat Fat, 0 g Trans Fat, 0 mg Chol, 110 mg Sod, 34g Total Carb, 11 g Total Sugar, 4 g Fib, 6 g Prot, 64 mg Calc

Minted Tabbouleh with bulgur and Persian cucumbers

If you are cooking in Summer, use 2 tomatoes instead of 1, because tomatoes more the most flavorful.

Ingredients (4 serves):

Bulgur	1 cup
Boiling water	1 cup
Large tomato, halved, seeded, and chopped	1
Mini (Persian) cucumbers, diced	2
Celery stalks, diced	2
Chopped fresh mint	½ cup
Chopped fresh parsley	½ cup
Lemon juice	1 tablespoon
Extra-virgin olive oil	1 tablespoon
Ground cumin	2 teaspoons
Salt	½ teaspoon
Black pepper	⅛ teaspoon

Directions:

1. Put the bulgur into a bowl and pour it with boiling water, then let it stand for about 30 minutes until the water is completely absorbed.

2. All the remaining ingredients should be added to bulgur and mixed very thoroughly. Transfer the finished salad to a salad bowl and serve to the table.

Per serving (about ½ cup): 223 grams, 181 Cal, 4 g Total Fat, 1 g Sat Fat, 0 g Trans Fat, 0 mg Chol, 338 mg Sod, 33 g Total Carb, 2 g Total Sugar, 9 g Fib, 6 g Prot, 72 mg Calc.

Salmon Salad with Horseradish

Ingredients (4 serves):

Small white potatoes, scrubbed	1¼ pound
Salmon fillet, skinned	1 (¾-pound)
Cold water	½ cup
Yellow bell pepper, diced	1
Dill pickle, thinly sliced	1
Snipped fresh chives	¼ cup
Plain fat-free yogurt	¾ cup
Prepared horseradish, drained	3 tablespoons
Reduced-fat mayonnaise	3 tablespoons
Salt	½ teaspoon
Lightly packed baby arugula	2 cups

Directions:

1. Peel the potatoes and wash under running water. Then put in a large saucepan, pour the water to cover the potatoes by 1 inch and bring them to a boil over medium heat.

2. Reduce the heat, cover with a lid and cook for about 12 minutes until the potatoes become soft.

3. Remove the potatoes and put them in a bowl to cool. Dice potatoes after it is cooled.

4. Meanwhile, take the salmon and rinse it in running cold water. Put it in a large saucepan, pour the water and bring to a boil. Reduce the temperature a little and cook it for about 8 minutes until the broth becomes clear. Get the salmon out with slotted spoon and put it on the plate to cool.

5. Grind the salmon fillet with a fork and mix with the potatoes, chives, bell paper and pickle in a large bowl.

6. To prepare a dressing for a salad, whisk in a blender yogurt, mayonnaise, horseradish, and salt. Line platter with arugula, then lettuce and evenly add the dressing on top.

Per serving (generous 1 cup salmon salad with ½ cup arugula): 339 grams, 317 Cal, 7 g Total Fat, 1 g Sat Fat, 0 g Trans Fat, 53 mg Chol, 725 mg Sod, 39 g Total Carb, 7 g Total Sugar, 4 g Fib, 24 g Prot, 114 mg Calc.

Salad Niçoise with Anchovy Fillets

Ingredients (6 serves):

Small red potatoes, scrubbed	1¼ pound
Trimmed green beans	2 cups
Large Boston or butter lettuce leaves	6
Lightly packed sliced romaine lettuce	4 cups
Water-packed light tuna drained and flaked	2 (5-ounce) cans
Cherry tomatoes, halved	24
Hard-cooked large eggs, peeled and quartered	2
Large pitted black olives, sliced	6
Anchovy fillets, rinsed and patted dry	4
Red wine vinegar	2 tablespoons
Lemon juice	2 tablespoons
Olive oil	1 tablespoon
Salt	¼ teaspoon
Black pepper	¼ teaspoon

Directions:

1. Peel the potatoes, rinse them under cold water and put them in a large saucepan. Fill with enough water, so that the water covers the potatoes by 1 inch and bring to a boil.

2. Reduce the temperature and cook for about 12 minutes until the potatoes become soft. Using a slotted spoon, take the potatoes out of the pan and cool them under running water. Then cut the potatoes into 4 pieces.

3. Add peas to the pot with water where the potatoes were boiled and cook for about 6 minutes until it becomes soft. Drain the water from the pan and rinse it under running water.

4. Lay the lettuce leaves on a dish and spread the potatoes, green peas, tomatoes, tuna and on top of the egg.

5. Evenly lay the olives and put the anchovy fillet on top.

6. To make a salad dressing, mix all the remaining ingredients in a small bowl, stir and add to the salad.

Per serving (about 3 caps): 502 grams, 362 Cal, 11 g Total Fat, 2 g Sat Fat, 0 g Trans Fat, 139 mg Chol, 673 mg Sod, 41 g Total Carb, 7 g Total Sugar, 7 g Fib, 27 g Prot, 103 mg Calc.

California Greens Salad with Baked Goat Cheese

Ingredients (6 serves):

Garlic clove, peeled	1
Salt	½ teaspoon
Extra-virgin olive oil	1 tablespoon
Lemon juice	1 tablespoon
Chopped fresh flat-leaf parsley	1 tablespoon
Small shallot, minced	1
Dijon mustard	1 teaspoon
Black pepper	¼ teaspoon
Plain dried bread crumbs	3 tablespoons
Finely ground walnuts	2 tablespoons
Reduced-fat soft goat cheese, cut into 6 rounds	2 ounces
Large egg white, lightly beaten	1
Lightly packed mixed baby salad greens	6 cups

Directions:

1. Preheat the oven to 400 ° F. Spray the pan evenly over the entire area and warm it in the oven.

2. Take a large kitchen knife and flatten the garlic on a cutting board. Then add salt and mash until smooth.

3. Use the container for the blender to prepare the dressing for the salad. Put the olive oil, parsley, lemon juice, shallots, pepper, garlic paste and mustard in it.

4. Using a blender mix all the ingredients.

5. Mix together walnuts and crumbs on waxed paper. Then, evenly stir the eggs and cheese and mix with the mixture of nuts.

6. Spread evenly throughout the pan and bake for about 5 minutes until all ingredients warm up.

7. In the meantime, rinse the lettuce leaves under cold water and put in a salad bowl. Add the dressing at the top of the salad and mix. Divide evenly the salad into 6 plates and put a warm goat cheese on top.

Per serving (1 salad) 89 grams, 75 Cal, 5 g Total Fat, 1 g Sat Fat, 0 g Trans Fat, 2 mg Chol, 309 mg Sod, 6 g Total Carb, 1 g Total Sugar, 1 g Fib, 3 g Prot, 48 mg Calc.

SOUPS—STARTERS and MAIN DISHES

Chilled Cucumber-Yogurt Soup

To cook a soup with more saturated and bright color add the tomatoes cut into cubes.

Ingredients (4 serves):

English (seedless) cucumbers, peeled	2
Container plain fat-free yogurt	1 (16-ounce)
Cmall garlic clove	1
Lemon juice	2 teaspoons
Salt	½ teaspoon
Black pepper	⅛ teaspoon
Scallions, sliced	2
lightly packed fresh mint leaves, finely chopped	½ cup

Directions:

1. Dice the cucumber about 1/3 cup, and cut the remaining quantity in larger pieces.

2. Blend the mix of lemon juice, garlic, yogurt, pepper, salt and cucumber slices.

3. Add onion and mint and again grind with a blender.

3. Pour everything into a large bowl and mix with the cucumber cubes.

4. Cover the pan with a lid and put the salad in the refrigerator for about 4 hours or overnight.

Per serving (generous 1 cup): 249 grams, 72 Cal, 0 g Total Fat, 0 g Sat Fat, 0 g Trans Fat, 3 mg Chol, 363 mg Sod, 14 g Total Carb, 8 g Total Sugar, 2 g Fib, 7 g Prot, 179 mg Calc.

French Onion Soup

The main secret of this dish is the very slow onion saute so that he could completely caramelize and get a dark golden color. It is a long cooking on a slow fire that can fully reveal the rich aroma of the dish.

Ingredients (4 serves):

Olive oil	2 teaspoons
Onions, thinly sliced	6
Sugar	1 teaspoon
Water	3 cups
Can reduced-sodium beef broth	1 (14½-ounce)
Salt	¼ teaspoon
Black pepper	¼ teaspoon
French bread, toasted	4 (1-ounce) slices
Shredded Gruyere cheese	$1/3$ cup

Directions:

1. Preheat a large skillet with oil over a medium heat. Add chopped onions and sprinkle with sugar. Then sauté onion for about 45 minutes stirring constantly until it turns dark golden.

2. Mix the chopped onions, broth, bell pepper, salt and add a little water. Bring to a boil, reduce heat, cover with a lid and cook for about 20 minutes.

3. Preheat the oven.

4. Put 4 flameproof bowls on the baking sheet. Pour soup into bowls, put a piece of bread on the top of each bowl and sprinkle with grated cheese Gruyere.

5. Bake for about 2 minutes until the cheese is melted.

Per serving (1 bowl): 480 grams, 175 Cal, 6 g Total Fat, 2 g Sat Fat, 0 g Trans Fat, 10 mg Chol, 468 mg Sod, 25 g Total Carb, 12 g Total Sugar, 4 g Fib, 7 g Prot, 140 mg Calc.

Creamy Yellow Squash Soup with Chives

Double celery and onion and cook for more 2 minutes.

Ingredients (4 serves):

olive oil	2 teaspoons
onion, chopped	1
celery stalk, chopped	1
garlic cloves, minced	2
yellow squash or zucchini, thinly	sliced 4
reduced-sodium chicken broth	1½ cups
salt	¼ teaspoon
black pepper	¼ teaspoon
fat-free sour cream	½ cup
snipped fresh chives	2 tablespoons

Directions:

1. Add oil in a large saucepan and heat it over medium heat. Then add the garlic and onions and fry until softened for about 5 minutes.

2. Add the squash, salt, pepper, and broth in a saucepan and bring to a boil. Then reduce the temperature and cook for about 15 minutes.

3 Using a blender, grind all the components of the soup. Pour the resulting puree soup into a large saucepan and cover with a lid. Then let the soup cool for at least 4 hours in the refrigerator.

4 Before serving the soup, add sour cream to the plate, and after pouring the soup, sprinkle with green chives.

Per serving (about 1 cup): 376 grams, 115 Cal, 3 g Total Fat, 1 g Sat Fat, 0 g Trans Fat, 3 mg Chol, 420 mg Sod, 19 g Total Carb, 9 g Total Sugar, 5 g Fib, 6 g Prot, 102 mg Calc.

Fresh Tomato-Basil Soup

Mind that the vegetable broth should be reduced-sodium one.

Ingredients (6 serves):

Extra-virgin olive oil	2 teaspoons
Chopped shallots	½ cup
Large tomatoes, coarsely chopped	4
Reduced-sodium vegetable broth	1 cup
Dried oregano	½ teaspoon
Salt	½ teaspoon
Black pepper	¼ teaspoon
Fat-free milk	2 cups
Tomato paste	¼ cup
Fat-free half-and-half	1 cup
Thinly sliced fresh basil	¼ cup

Directions:

1. Preheat the saucepan with oil over medium heat and add shallot onion, cook it for about 5 minutes, until it is softened. Then add the tomatoes, oregano, broth, pepper, and salt and bring to a boil.

2. Reduce the temperature and simmer for about 6 minutes until the tomatoes become softened, then remove the pan from the plate and let it cool for about 5 minutes.

3. Grind all the ingredients in a blender.

4. Mix tomato paste and a glass of milk until smooth in a small bowl. Add the resulting milk to the soup and another glass of milk, as well as basil.

5. Then at medium temperature, heat the soup for about 5 minutes. Do not bring it to a boil.

Per serving (about 1 cup): 311 grams, 120 Cal, 2 g Total Fat, 0 g Sat Fat, 0 g Trans Fat, 2 mg Chol, 366 mg Sod, 19 g Total Carb, 12 g Total Sugar, 2 g Fib, 6 g Prot, 174 mg Calc.

Butternut Squash and Sage Soup

You need to peel and core 1 large Granny Smith's apple, dice it and add with squash in step 2.

Ingredients (4 serves):

Butternut squash, peeled, seeded, and cut into 2-inch chunks	1 (2½- to 3-pound)
Olive oil	1 tablespoon
Onion, chopped	1
Large leek (white and pale green parts only), sliced	1
Garlic cloves, minced	2
Reduced-sodium vegetable broth	3 cups
Dried sage, crumbled	1½ teaspoons
Black pepper	¼ teaspoon

Directions:

1. Put a squash in steamer container, pour water and bring to a boil. Cook for about 15 minutes until the squash becomes soft and at the same time retains its shape.

2. Meanwhile, heat the oil over medium heat in a large saucepan. Add the leeks, garlic, and onions and cook about 5 minutes until softened.

3. Then transfer the squash into a saucepan, add all the remaining ingredients and bring to a boil.

4. Reduce the temperature and stew for about 15 minutes with the lid on, until the squash becomes even softer.

5. Remove the pan from the plate and let it cool for about 5 minutes.

6. Use a blender to make a pureed soup, and then reheat the soup at medium temperature.

Per serving (about 1½ cups): 487 grams, 192 Cal, 4 g Total Fat, 1 g Sat Fat, 0 g Trans Fat, 0 mg Chol, 366 mg Sod, 39 g Total Carb, 12 g Total Sugar, 10 g Fib, 4 g Prot, 158 mg Calc.

Potato-Watercress Soup

Leek tends to hold some sand and dirt between layers and it is important to wash everything thoroughly.

Ingredients (6 serves):

all-purpose potatoes, peeled and cut into ½-inch pieces	4
leeks (white and pale green part only), sliced	2
large onion, chopped	1
reduced-sodium chicken broth	4½ cups
black pepper	¼ teaspoon
watercress, trimmed	½ bunch
fat-free half-and-half	½ cup

Directions:

1. Mix the leeks, broth, potatoes, and peppers in a large saucepan and bring to a boil.

2. Reduce the temperature, cover with a lid and stew for about 20 minutes.

2. Add the watercress to the soup and continue to simmer for about 5 minutes until the potatoes and watercress are softened. Then remove the pan from the stove.

3. To create a cream soup, blend the soup in a blender and reheat over medium heat.

Per serving (1⅓ cups): 349 grams, 133 Cal, 0 g Total Fat, 0 g Sat Fat, 0 g Trans Fat, 0 mg Chol, 496 mg Sod, 28 g Total Carb, 6 g Total Sugar, 3 g Fib, 6 g Prot, 61 mg Calc.

Food Processor Gazpacho

There is a wonderful and very convenient way to remove the skin from a tomato. At the base of the tomato, make a cross-cut × and place in a bowl with boiling water for 1 minute. Then take the tomato with a tablespoon and put it in a bowl with cold water for a minute. Then peel tomatoes.

Ingredients (4 serves):

Plum tomatoes, peeled and sliced	4
Cucumber, peeled, seeded, and coarsely chopped	½
Red bell pepper, cut into chunks	½
Scallions, sliced	4
Garlic clove, minced	1
Red wine vinegar	2 tablespoons
Tomato juice, chilled	2 cups
Black pepper	¼ teaspoon
Hot sauce	few drops
Diced cucumber	¼ cup
Diced red bell pepper	¼ cup
Diced red onion	¼ cup

Directions:

1. Mix cucumber, sweet pepper, tomatoes, garlic, onion and vinegar in a bowl for a blender and mix in the puree.

2. Then pour into a large saucepan and add the tomato juice, hot sauce, and black pepper. Cover with a lid and let cool for at least 4 hours or overnight.

3. Spread gazpacho on 4 chilled bowls and put on top diced pepper, onions and cucumber.

Per serving (¼ of soup): 272 grams, 60 Cal, 0 g Total Fat, 0 g Sat Fat, 0 g Trans Fat, 0 mg Chol, 441 mg Sod, 12 g Total Carb, 7 g Total Sugar, 3 g Fib, 2 g Prot, 33 mg Calc.

Chinese Noodle Soup

To save time, order roasted pork at one of the local Chinese restaurants to use in this soup.

Ingredients (6 serves):

Carton reduced-sodium chicken	1 (48-ounce)
Scallions, sliced on diagonal	2
Fresh ginger, peeled and minced	1 (1-inch) piece
Reduced-sodium soy sauce	1 tablespoon
Baby bok choy, halved	6
Matchstick-cut carrots	1 cup
Cooked whole wheat capellini	2 cups
Lean cooked pork, cut into matchsticks	6 ounces
Lightly packed baby spinach	1 cup

Directions:

1. Mix the broth, soy sauce, ginger, and onions in a large saucepan and bring to a boil. Cook for about 3 minutes until the scallions become soft.

2. Add carrots and bok choy and cook about 7 minutes at a low temperature.

3. Mix pasta, fried pork, and spinach with the soup and cook at medium temperature for about 2 minutes until the spinach is wilted.

Per serving (1½ cups): 369 grams, 137 Cal, 2 g Total Fat, 1 g Sat Fat, 0 g Trans Fat, 823 mg Chol, 743 mg Sod, 17 g Total Carb, 3 g Total Sugar, 3 g Fib, 15 g Prot, 52 mg Calc.

Bok Choy–Noodle Soup

The so-called glass noodles are made from ground beans. After it is properly soaked and cooked, it becomes translucent.

Ingredients (6 serves):

Cellophane noodles	4 ounces
Reduced-sodium chicken broth	2 (14½-ounce) cans
Low-fat extra-firm tofu, cut into ½-inch dice	1 (12-ounce) package
Baby bok choy, coarsely chopped	½ pound
Watercress, trimmed	½ bunch
Scallions, thinly sliced on diagonal	2
Reduced-sodium soy sauce	2 tablespoons
Asian (dark) sesame oil	1 teaspoon
Black pepper	½ teaspoon

Directions:

1. Pre-boil the water in the pan and put the noodles in it, so that the water covers it and let it stand for about 10 minutes until the noodles become soft.

2. Then drain the water and cut the noodles with 3-inch strips with kitchen scissors.

3. Mix broth, bok choy, watercress and tofu into a large saucepan and to bring to a boil. Then cook for about 5 minutes until the vegetables become tender.

4. Add the noodles, soy sauce, sesame oil, onion, and pepper and cook for about 2 minutes.

Per serving (1 cup): 266 grams, 123 Cal, 2 g Total Fat, 0 g Sat Fat, 0 g Trans Fat, 0 mg Chol, 617 mg Sod, 20 g Total Carb, 1 g Total Sugar, 1 g Fib, 7 g Prot, 67 mg Calc.

Creamy Bean Soup

To prepare the soup, you can successfully use almost any canned beans. For admirers of chunkier soup, we advise to knead beans with a fork, and not grind them in the puree.

Ingredients (6 serves):

Cannellini (white kidney) beans, rinsed and drained	1 (15½-ounce) can
Chickpeas, rinsed and drained	1 (15½-ounce) can
Reduced-sodium vegetable broth	3 cups
Olive oil	2 teaspoons
Onion, chopped	1
Garlic cloves, minced	2
Fat-free half-and-half	½ cup
Grated Parmesan cheese	¼ cup
Black pepper	⅛ teaspoon

Directions:

1. Pour ½ cup of broth into the blender container, put cannellini beans and chickpeas and mix everything in the puree.

2. Preheat a large saucepan with oil. Then add onions and garlic and fry for about 5 minutes until soft.

3. Pour in the remaining 2½ cups of broth and add the beans puree. Bring the soup to a boil stirring from time to time.

4. Add pepper and Parmesan and bring to a boil again at medium temperature.

Per serving (1¼ cups): 400 grams, 219 Cal, 5 g Total Fat, 1 g Sat Fat, 0 g Trans Fat, 4 mg Chol, 665 mg Sod, 31 g Total Carb, 8 g Total Sugar, 7 g Fib, 11 g Prot, 186 mg Calc.

Creamy Corn, Potato, and Bacon Soup

Turn this super-delicious and super-easy soup into chowder and live it chunky.

Ingredients (4 serves):

Olive oil	2 teaspoons
Onion, chopped	1
Yellow bell pepper, chopped	½
All-purpose potatoes, peeled and diced	1 pound
Reduced-sodium chicken broth	2½ cups
Fresh or thawed frozen corn kernels	2 cups
Fat-free half-and-half	¼ cup
Turkey bacon, crisp cooked and cut into ½-inch pieces	2 slices
Snipped fresh chives	2 tablespoons

Directions:

1. Pre-heat the oil in a large saucepan at medium temperature. Pour the bell pepper and onion and fry for about 5 minutes until soft.

2. Add the broth and potatoes and bring to a boil. Reduce the heat, cover it with a lid and cook for about 10 minutes until the potatoes become soft.

3. Add the sweet corn and let it simmer for about 5 minutes. After put the saucepan form away from heat.

4. Use a blender to make puree soup. Then stir the soup and heat again over medium heat.

5. Pour the soup into 4 bowls and sprinkle chives and bacon.

Per serving (about 1¼ cups): 365 grams, 250 Cal, 4 g Total Fat, 0 g Sat Fat, 0 g Trans Fat, 6 mg Chol, 505 mg Sod, 47 g Total Carb, 7 g Total Sugar, 5 g Fib, 9 g Prot, 40 mg Calc.

African Peanut Soup

Adding fresh ginger gives a special spicy taste in this soup. If you like the taste of ginger, you can replace a ½ teaspoon of dry ginger with fresh.

Ingredients (4 serves):

Chickpeas, rinsed and drained	1 (15½-ounce) can
Reduced-sodium vegetable broth	3 cups
Creamy peanut butter	3 tablespoons
Onions, chopped	2
Fresh ginger, peeled and minced	1 (1-inch) piece
Curry powder	2 teaspoons
Diced tomatoes	1 (14½-ounce) can
Tomato paste	1 tablespoon
Cayenne	¼ teaspoon
Chopped fresh cilantro	¼ cup
Scallions, thinly sliced	2

Directions:

1. Add ½ cup of broth, peanut butter and chickpeas into the blender container and mix in the puree.

2. Preheat a large non-stick saucepan at medium temperature and add ginger and onion to it. Fry stirring for about 5 minutes until the onion is tender.

3. Add the curry and cook for about a minute. Pour the remaining broth and put the tomatoes, chickpeas puree, tomato paste, cayenne and bring to a boil.

4. Then reduce the heat and cook for about 5 minutes so that all the ingredients reveal their taste.

5. Pour the soup into 4 bowls and sprinkle with scallions and cilantro.

Per serving (about 1½ cups): 460 grams, 217 Cal, 8 g Total Fat, 1 g Sat Fat, 0 g Trans Fat, 0 mg Chol, 664 mg Sod, 30 g Total Carb, 13 g Total Sugar, 8 g Fib, 9 g Prot, 85 mg Calc.

Lentil and Swiss Chard Soup

To give the soup a brighter flavor in the first stage of cooking (step 1) add 14½ ounces of dried tomatoes.

Ingredients (4 serves):

olive oil	2 teaspoons
onion, chopped	1
garlic clove, minced	1
dried brown lentils, picked over, rinsed, and drained	1 cup
reduced-sodium vegetable broth	4 cups
lightly packed thinly sliced Swiss chard leaves	2 cups
salt	¼ teaspoon
black pepper	1/8 teaspoon
lemon juice	2 teaspoons

Directions:

1. Preheat a large saucepan, add oil and heat as well. Add garlic, onion and cook about 5 minutes before softening.

2. Add broth and lentils and bring to a boil. Cook covered with a lid for about 45 minutes until the lentils become soft.

3. Add the Swiss chard, pepper, and salt in the soup and cook stirring for about 5 minutes until the chard is softened. Then add the lemon juice.

Per serving (about 1½ cups): 436 grams, 216 Cal, 3 g Total Fat, 0 g Sat Fat, 0 g Trans Fat, 0 mg Chol, 799 mg Sod, 34 g Total Carb, 6 g Total Sugar, 12 g Fib, 16 g Prot, 46 mg Calc.

Classic Beef-Barley Soup

Increase the number of celery stalks and carrots to 3 each.

Ingredients (4 serves):

round steak, trimmed and cut into ½-inch pieces	½ pound
pearl barley	½ cup
water	5 cups
onion, chopped	1
carrots, diced	2
celery stalks, diced	2
salt	1 teaspoon
black pepper	1/8 teaspoon
frozen baby lima beans, thawed	1 cup
sliced white or cremini mushrooms	2 cups

Directions:

1. Pour the pan with water bring it to a boil and then add the steak and barley. The foam that will be formed on the surface should be removed with a slotted spoon.

2. Add carrots, celery, onion, and peppers. Slightly reduce the heat, cover and cook for about 30 minutes.

2. Add the mushrooms and lima beans to the broth and cook for about 15 minutes until the meat becomes tender.

Per serving (about 2 cups): 532 grams, 180 Cal, 2 g Total Fat, 1 g Sat Fat, 0 g Trans Fat, 29 mg Chol, 665 mg Sod, 24 g Total Carb, 7 g Total Sugar, 6 g Fib, 17 g Prot, 51 mg Calc.

Smoky Manhattan-Style Clam Chowder

In order not to toughen calms do not boil them in step 2.

Ingredients (4 serves):

olive oil	2 teaspoons
onion, chopped	1
large garlic clove, minced	1
all-purpose potato, peeled and cut into ½-inch dice	1 (½-pound)
small zucchini, diced	1
celery stalk, diced	1
carrot, diced	1
pre-roasted diced tomatoes	1 (14½-ounce) can
clam juice	2 (8-ounce) bottles
water	½ cup
dried oregano	½ teaspoon
black pepper	⅛ teaspoons
chopped clams	1 (6½-ounce) can

Directions:

1. Preheat a large saucepan at medium temperature and pour oil. Then add the garlic and onions and fry them for about 5 minutes until the onion is tender enough.

2. Add zucchini, carrots, potatoes, celery and cook for about 5 minutes stirring.

3. Add the clam juice, tomatoes with the juice, pepper, and oregano and bring to a boil.

4. Reduce the temperature, cover and cook for about 15 minutes. Add clams with juice and cook them for no more than 2 minutes stirring.

Per serving (1½ cups): 417 grams, 143 Cal, 3 g Total Fat, 0 g Sat Fat, 0 g Trans Fat, 16 mg Chol, 657 mg Sod, 22 g Total Carb, 8 g Total Sugar, 4 g Fib, 9 g Prot, 61 mg Calc.

BEEF, PORK, and LAMB

Peppered Roast Tenderloin Trimmed and Tied

Crush the peppercorns with a mortar and wrap in a clean kitchen towel, well mash with a meat hammer or heavy frying pan.

Ingredients (10 serves):

Beef tenderloin, trimmed and tied	1 (2½-pound)
Garlic cloves, thinly sliced lengthwise	2
Olive oil	4 teaspoons
Cracked black peppercorns	1 tablespoon
Finely chopped fresh rosemary	2 teaspoons
Finely chopped fresh thyme	2 teaspoons
Finely chopped fresh sage	2 teaspoons
Salt	½ teaspoon

Directions:

1. Preheat the oven to 425 ° F.

2. Using a thin knife, make small in-depth dimensions along the entire length of the tenderloin and insert a piece of garlic in each cut and rub the whole piece of meat with oil. 3. To make the seasoning for meat, mix the rosemary, peppercorns, sage, thyme, and salt in a cup, and then evenly apply to the meat.

4. Put the tenderloin on a baking sheet and put in the oven for about 10 minutes and then reduce the temperature to 350 ° F.

5. Cook the meat for about 20 minutes, periodically checking the internal temperature of the meat with an instant-read thermometer until the temperature reaches 145 ° F.

6. After put the meat on a cutting board and let it stand for about 15 minutes. Then cut into 15-20 even slices.

Per serving (2 slices): 89 grams, 183 Cal, 9 g Total Fat, 3 g Sat Fat, 0 g Trans Fat, 67 mg Chol, 167 mg Sod, 1 g Total Carb, 0 g Total Sugar, 0 g Fib, 24 g Prot, 21 mg Calc.

Grilled T-Bone Steak

Mix together a tomato-corn salad made from 2 cups of sweet corn and several grape tomatoes cut in half and finely chopped red onion seasoned with lemon juice and a pinch of salt.

Ingredients (4 serves):

Finely chopped fresh rosemary	2 teaspoons
Finely chopped fresh sage	2 teaspoons
Olive oil	1 teaspoon
Salt	½ teaspoon
Black pepper	¼ teaspoon
T-bone or rib steak, about 1-inch-thick, trimmed	1 (1¼-pound)

Directions:

1. Preheat the grill rack and spray with a nonstick spray and if you are using direct-method, heat the grate with medium fire.

2. To prepare rub, mix all the ingredients together in a bowl, except the steak. Then, season the steak on both sides and place on the grill.

3. Fry the steak for about 5 minutes on each side, regularly check the temperature inside the steak until the instant-read thermometer shows 145 ° F.

4. Put the steak on the cutting board and after 5 minutes, cut into 4 pieces.

Per serving (¼ of steak): 109 grams, 213 Cal, 11 g Total Fat, 3 g Sat Fat, 0 g Trans Fat, 58 mg Chol, 366 mg Sod, 0 g Total Carb, 0 g Total Sugar, 0 g Fib, 28 g Prot, 8 mg Calc.

Dry Red Wine London Broil

Serve the plate for the dish with potatoes and broccoli steamed.

Ingredients (4 serves):

Dry red wine 1 garlic clove, minced	½ cup
Chopped fresh rosemary	1 tablespoon
Salt	½ teaspoon
Black pepper	¼ teaspoon
Top round or sirloin tip steak, trimmed	1 (1-pound)

Directions:

1. Mix together the wine, rosemary, garlic, pepper, and salt in a large zip plastic bag and put the meat into it. Squeeze the air out of the bag and put it in the refrigerator and refrigerate for 6 hours to up 1 day sometimes turning the bag over.

2. Preheat the oven and broiler well.

3. Take the steak from the bag and remove the marinade from the meat surface. Then put the steak on broiler rack and fry for about 4 minutes on each side.

4. Using an instant-read thermometer, measure the temperature inside the steak and when it reaches 145 ° F, the steak is ready.

5.Transfer the meat to a cutting board and leave for 5 minutes. Cut the steak into 16 slices.

Per serving (4 slices): 117 grams, 186 Cal, 5 g Total Fat, 2 g Sat Fat, 0 g Trans Fat, 56 mg Chol, 327 mg Sod, 1 g Total Carb, 0 g Total Sugar, 0 g Fib, 27 g Prot, 12 mg Calc.

Soy Sauce Marinated Flank Steak

To master a stalk of lemongrass, cut the thin upper half of the stalk. Clean the dry leaves from the bulbous stalk, leaving tender inner leaves only and chop the stalk.

Ingredients (4 serves):

Reduced-sodium soy sauce	¼ cup
Dry sherry	2 tablespoons
Honey	1 tablespoon
Grated peeled fresh ginger	1 tablespoon
Finely chopped lemongrass	1 tablespoon
Garlic cloves, minced	1 tablespoon
Red pepper flakes	1 pinch
Flank steak, trimmed	1 (1-pound)
Olive oil	2 teaspoons
Black pepper	¼ teaspoon

Directions:

1. Mix the sherry, honey, soy sauce, ginger, lemongrass, pepper flakes and garlic in a zip-close plastic bag and put the steak inside.

2. Remove excess air and close it. Put the package in the refrigerator to cool from 4 hours to 1 day and periodically turn it over.

3. Preheat the oven and the broiler.

4. Get the steak from the bag and remove the marinade from the surface of the meat. Wipe the steak with a dry towel and then rub it with oil on both sides and season with black melted pepper.

5. Put the steak on a broiler and fry for about 5 minutes on each side. Be sure to use the instant-read thermometer and check the temperature inside the steak. Once the temperature reaches 145 ° F, the steak is ready.

6. Put the steak on the chopping board and leave for 5 minutes. Slice it across grain into 12 pieces.

Per serving (3 slices): 123 grams, 219 Cal, 9 g Total Fat, 3 g Sat Fat, 0 g Trans Fat, 42 mg Chol, 530 mg Sod, 8 g Total Carb, 4 g Total Sugar, 0 g Fib, 25 g Prot, 21 mg Calc.

Our Favorite Meat Loaf with White Mushrooms

For thoroughly cooked (well done) bake 30–45 minutes longer.

Ingredients (4 serves):

Canola oil	2 teaspoons
Finely chopped white mushrooms	1 cup
Onion, finely chopped	1
Carrot, finely chopped	1
Celery stalk, finely chopped	1
Lean ground beef (7% fat or less)	1 pound
Quick-cooking (not instant) oats	½ cup
Large egg whites	2
Ketchup	3 tablespoons
Worcestershire sauce	1 tablespoon
Finely chopped fresh thyme	2 teaspoons
Salt	¼ teaspoon
Black pepper	¼ teaspoon
Garlic cloves, minced	1
Tomato puree or tomato sauce	¼ cup

Directions:

1. Preheat the oven to 350 ° F.

2. Heat the oil in a frying pan over medium heat and add the celery, onions, mushrooms, and carrots. Fry stirring for about 5 minutes until the onion is soft.

3. Then put everything in a large bowl.

4. Mix all the other ingredients and vegetables in a bowl, except tomato puree. Mix the minced meat and other ingredients thoroughly and put it into a 4½ × 8½-inch loaf pan.

5. After shaping the meatloaf, spread it with tomato paste on top, put in the oven and bake for about 30 minutes.

6. Using an instant-read thermometer, check the temperature of the meat and as soon as the value is 160 ° F the meatloaf is ready.

7. Remove it from the oven and let it stand for about 5 minutes. Cut into slices.

Per serving (2 slices): 193 grams, 243 Cal, 8 g Total Fat, 3 g Sat Fat, 0 g Trans Fat, 59 mg Chol, 421 mg Sod, 15 g Total Carb, 5 g Total Sugar, 2 g Fib, 26 g Prot, 35 mg Calc.

Red Wine Beef Stew with fresh mint

Discard mint and parsley bay leaf with kitchen scissors.

Ingredients (4 serves):

Olive oil	2 teaspoons
Beef round, cut into 1½-inch chunks	1 pound
Onion, chopped	1
Diced tomatoes	1 (14½-ounce) can
Reduced-sodium beef broth	1 cup
Dry red wine	½ cup
Dried thyme	½ teaspoon
Salt	½ teaspoon
Black pepper	¼ teaspoon
Bay leaf	1
Frozen pearl onions	16
Carrots, cut into 1-inch chunks	4
Potatoes, peeled and cut into 1-inch chunks	4
Frozen green peas	1 cup
Chopped fresh flat-leaf parsley	1 tablespoon
Chopped fresh mint	1 tablespoon

Directions:

1. Heat the oil in a Dutch oven over medium heat and add chopped beef. Fry the meat stirring until it becomes brownish golden on all sides.

2. Transfer the meat to a plate. Add the onions to the pot and fry for about 5 minutes until it becomes soft.

3. Put the meat back into the pot again. Add the broth, tomatoes with juice, wine, salt, thyme, bay leaf and pepper to the pot and bring to a boil.

4. Then reduce the temperature and cook stirring for about 45 minutes, partially covered.

5. Add carrots, potatoes and pearl onions to the pot and cook for about 30 minutes. After add peas, stir and cook for about 10 minutes. At the end, add fresh parsley and mint.

Per serving (about 2 cups): 441 grams, 426 Cal, 10 g Total Fat, 2 g Sat Fat, 0 g Trans Fat, 59 mg Chol, 460 mg Sod, 57 g Total Carb, 13 g Total Sugar, 8 g Fib, 27 g Prot, 60 mg Calc.

Beef and Bean Chili

Serve the plate with sour cream and rice.

Ingredients (6 serves):

olive oil	2 teaspoons
large onion, chopped	1
carrots, chopped	2
celery stalks, chopped	2
red bell pepper, chopped	1
large garlic cloves, minced	3
lean ground beef (7% fat or less)	1 pound
chili powder	1 tablespoon
ground cumin	2 teaspoons
dried oregano	½ teaspoon
salt	½ teaspoon
black pepper	¼ teaspoon
fire-roasted diced tomatoes	1 (14½-ounce) can
red kidney beans, rinsed and drained	1 (15½-ounce) can
fat-free sour cream	6 tablespoons
hot cooked brown rice	3 cups

Directions:

1. Pour the oil into a large Dutch oven and preheat it at medium temperature.

2.Add the carrots, celery, onions, garlic and bell peppers and fry about 15 minutes until the celery and carrots are soft.

3. Add the beef to the pot and fry for about 7 minutes stirring with a wooden spoon until it turns brown.

4. Add cumin, oregano, chili powder and black pepper and cook for about 2 minutes more.

5. Add the beans and tomatoes with the juice in the pot and bring to a boil and then reduce the temperature, partially cover with a lid and cook stirring for about 20 minutes.

Per serving (about 1½ cups chili, ½ cup rice, and 1 tablespoon sour cream): 396 grams, 373 Cal, 7 g Total Fat, 2 g Sat Fat, 0 g Trans Fat, 47 mg Chol, 452 mg Sod, 52 g Total Carb, 8 g Total Sugar, 11 g Fib, 25 g Prot, 83 mg Calc.

Buffalo Meat Cheddar-Stuffed Burgers

Buffalo meat, sometimes known as bison meat, is very fragrant and has less cholesterol and fat than beef.

Ingredients (4 serves):

Ground buffalo meat or lean ground beef (7% fat or less)	1 pound
Small Vidalia onion, finely chopped	1
Worcestershire sauce	1 teaspoon
Salt	½ teaspoon
Black pepper	⅛ teaspoon
Shredded reduced-fat Cheddar cheese	½ cup
English muffins, split and toasted	4
Thinly sliced romaine lettuce	1 cup
Small tomato slices	16

Directions:

1. Combine onion, buffalo, salt, Worcester-shire sauce and pepper in a large bowl. Wet your hands with cold water and make 4 identical round balls.

2. Finger a groove in each of them and fill the groove with 2 tablespoons of Cheddar. Close the filling by squeezing the meat. Then the balls should be shaped into ¾-inch patties.

3. Heat a large skillet and add some oil. Then put the meat patties and fry on both sides for about 4 minutes.

4. Be sure to measure the temperature inside with an instant-read thermometer and when the temperature is 145 ° F, the patties are ready.

5. Spread the bottom of the muffins on the plates and on top of each put lettuce, burgers, tomato slices and cover with the top of the muffins.

Per serving (1 garnished burger): 224 grams, 343 Cal, 12 g Total Fat, 5 g Sat Fat, 0 g Trans Fat, 70 mg Chol, 754 mg Sod, 30 g Total Carb, 2 g Total Sugar, 3 g Fib, 30 g Prot, 257 mg Calc.

Argentina-Style Steak and Sauce

Try to add more cold water to give the mixture a saucy consistency, if needed (in step 2).

Ingredients (4 serves):

Lightly packed fresh flat-leaf parsley leaves, chopped	1 cup
Lightly packed fresh cilantro leaves, chopped	½ cup
Red wine vinegar	1 tablespoon
Olive oil	1 tablespoon
Salt	½ teaspoon
Red pepper flakes	¼ teaspoon
Top round steak, trimmed	1 (1-pound)
Black pepper	¼ teaspoon

Directions:

1. Spray grill rack with oil and preheat.

2. To make the sauce, mix cilantro, parsley, oil, vinegar, pepper flakes and ¼ teaspoon of salt in a bowl.

3. Sprinkle the steak with black pepper and the remaining salt. Put the steak on the grill and fry about 6 minutes on each side.

4. Check the inside temperature of the steak with an instant-read thermometer and when the temperature is 145 ° F the steak is ready and it can be removed from the rack.

4. Put the steak on the chopping board and leave for 10 minutes.

5. Thinly cut the steak into 10-12 pieces and serve with sauce.

Per serving (about 3 slices steak and 1½ tablespoons sauce): 110 grams, 197 Cal, 9 g Total Fat, 2 g Sat Fat, 0 g Trans Fat, 65 mg Chol, 480 mg Sod, 2 g Total Carb, 0 g Total Sugar, 0 g Fib, 27 g Prot, 29 mg Calc.

Pork Roast with Winter Vegetables

Inserted instant-read thermometer registers 160°F – pork is medium rare.

Ingredients (8 serves):

Large garlic cloves, minced Grated zest of ½ lemon	2
Chopped fresh rosemary	1 tablespoon
Salt	1½ teaspoons
Black pepper	½ teaspoon
Boneless center-cut pork loin roast, trimmed	1 (2-pound)
Butternut squash, peeled, seeded, and cut into 16 pieces	½
Large parsnips, cut into 2-inch lengths	2
Large carrots, cut into 2-inch lengths	2
Celery stalks, cut into 2-inch lengths	4
Extra-virgin olive oil	4 teaspoons

Directions:

1. Preheat the oven to 450 ° F and spray the roasting pan with oil.

2. Mix the rosemary, lemon zest, garlic, ¼ teaspoon pepper and ¾ teaspoon of salt and rub the meat from all sides.

3. Put the meat in the oven. Lay parsnip, scatter squash, carrots around the meat and season with the remaining ¼ teaspoon of pepper and ¾ teaspoon of salt.

4. Fry the meat for about 45 minutes.

5. Put the pork on a cutting board and leave for 10 minutes. Then cut into 12-14 slices and serve the meat along with the vegetables.

Per serving (2 slices pork and 1 cup vegetables): 242 grams, 281 Cal, 14 g Total Fat, 5 g Sat Fat, 0 g Trans Fat, 68 mg Chol, 544 mg Sod, 14 g Total Carb, 4 g Total Sugar, 4 g Fib, 24 g Prot, 76 mg Calc.

Honey-Mustard Pork Chops

Serve these delightful chops with steamed sliced ears of corn and steamed fresh kale.

Ingredients (8 serves):

Dijon mustard 4 teaspoons honey	¼ cup
Cider or white wine vinegar	1 teaspoon
Black pepper	¼ teaspoon
Bone-in loin pork chops, about 1-inch thick	4 (5-ounce)

Directions:

1. To prepare the marinade, mix all ingredients except pork in a cup.

2. Transfer the marinade into a large plastic bag with a zipper and put the pork into it. Remove the air and close. Take the package to the refrigerator and cool from 4 hours to overnight.

3. Spray the frying pan with oil and heat over medium heat.

4. Take the chops from the package and remove the marinade from them.

5. Place the chops in the pan and fry for 6 minutes on each side.

Per serving (1 chop): 94 grams, 165 Cal, 5 g Total Fat, 2 g Sat Fat, 0 g Trans Fat, 59 mg Chol, 546 mg Sod, 9 g Total Carb, 5 g Total Sugar, 0 g Fib, 19 g Prot, 17 mg Calc.)

Spicy Pork Stir-Fry

Serve the plate with wild rice and fresh basil.

Ingredients (4 serves):

canola oil	2 teaspoons
Pork tenderloin, trimmed and thinly sliced	1-pound
Red bell pepper, cut into thick strips	1
Scallions, cut into 2-inch lengths	8
Pineapple chunks, drained	1 (20-ounce) can
Tomatoes, each cut into 8 wedges	2
Jalapeño pepper, seeded and minced	1
Grated peeled fresh ginger	2 teaspoons
Garlic cloves, minced	2
Soy sauce	4 teaspoons
Asian (dark) sesame oil	1 teaspoon
Chopped fresh cilantro	¼ cup
Hot cooked white rice	2 cups

Directions:

1. Preheat the wok pan at a very high temperature, add the canola oil and spread throughout the pan. Put the pork into a wok pan and fry 1-2 minutes on each side to make the meat pinkish. Then use the tongs to remove the meat and put it on the plate.

2. Get the bell pepper in the pan and fry it stirring for 2 minutes. Then add onion and cook for 2 more minutes.

3. Then put pineapple and simmer for another 30 seconds.

4. Lay out the pork and add ginger, garlic, jalapeño, sesame oil and soy sauce. Fry until all ingredients are warmed up, and then another 2 minutes.

5. Put it out the dish on a plate, sprinkle with fresh cilantro.

Per serving (about 1½ cups pork mixture and ½ cup rice): 430 grams, 419 Cal, 12 g Total Fat, 3 g Sat Fat, 0 g Trans Fat, 56 mg Chol, 491 mg Sod, 52 g Total Carb, 24 g Total Sugar, 4 g Fib, 27 g Prot, 81 mg Calc.

Conclusion

Dear reader, thank you for reading this book, hope that you are on your way to a healthy life and nothing can stop you in this effort. While you cook your next masterpiece according to our recipes and getting right to a set goal, thousands of people around the world who also become your like-minded also have chosen a healthy lifestyle and conquered new heights of culinary with our recipes.

Each of our readers is unique and has its own idea of delicious and healthy food. It does not actually matter whether it is a daily meal or an exquisite dinner. The main feature of this book will be a daily practice of choosing and cooking exactly the food that brings pleasure and also helps systematically to reduce your weight.

Soon you will be able to achieve a tangible effect by literally reducing the calorie content of food and thus achieving a calorie deficit obtained during the day. At the same time using our unique experience in weight reduction, you will achieve great results without any damage to taste preferences and lifestyle.

We also draw your attention to the fact that using the unique recipes you will be able to calculate your daily calorie points by yourself. Our recipes are based on the calorie content of food, protein and carbohydrate content. The uniqueness of this formula is that the precise number of these elements determined per day that will help your body to easily digest the food and gradually reduce weight. By tracking your results and counting daily calorie scores, you can easily lose weight and achieve the desired result.

Remember that weight loss should not be a tough process for you. With our recipes, this will be a wonderful and interesting journey into the world of delicious, varied and at the same time healthy food.

Author's Afterthoughts

Thanks ever so much to each of my cherished readers for investing the time read this book!

I know you could have picked from many other books but you chose this one. So big thanks for downloading this book and reading all way to the end.

If you enjoyed this book or received value from it, I'd like to ask you for a favor. Please take a few minutes to post an honest and heartfelt review on Amazon.com Your support does make a difference and to benefit other people.